YOUR KNOWLEDGE HAS VALUE

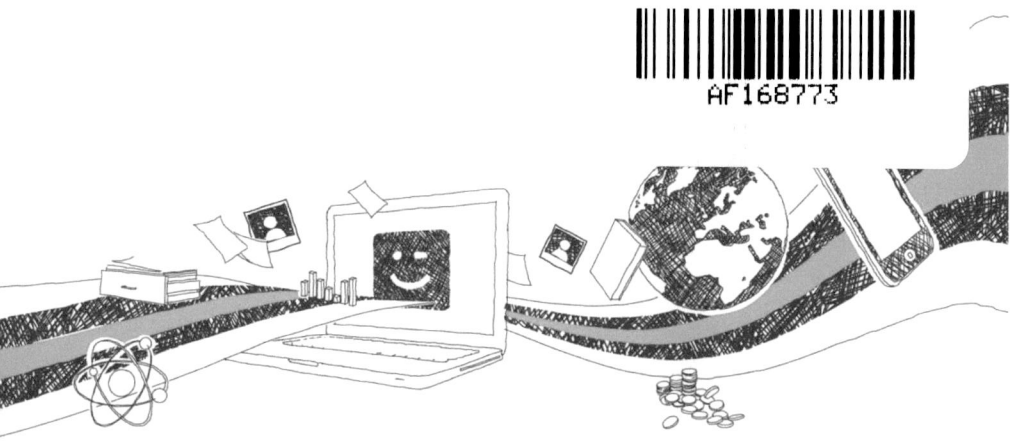

- We will publish your bachelor's and master's thesis, essays and papers

- Your own eBook and book -
  sold worldwide in all relevant shops

- Earn money with each sale

Upload your text at www.GRIN.com
and publish for free

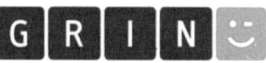

Bibliographic information published by the German National Library:

The German National Library lists this publication in the National Bibliography; detailed bibliographic data are available on the Internet at http://dnb.dnb.de .

This book is copyright material and must not be copied, reproduced, transferred, distributed, leased, licensed or publicly performed or used in any way except as specifically permitted in writing by the publishers, as allowed under the terms and conditions under which it was purchased or as strictly permitted by applicable copyright law. Any unauthorized distribution or use of this text may be a direct infringement of the author s and publisher s rights and those responsible may be liable in law accordingly.

Imprint:

Copyright © 2016 GRIN Verlag
Print and binding: Books on Demand GmbH, Norderstedt Germany
ISBN: 9783668726710

This book at GRIN:

https://www.grin.com/document/428453

Rodney Mulelu

Implementation of the ward based outreach teams programme in the rural area

GRIN Verlag

GRIN - Your knowledge has value

Since its foundation in 1998, GRIN has specialized in publishing academic texts by students, college teachers and other academics as e-book and printed book. The website www.grin.com is an ideal platform for presenting term papers, final papers, scientific essays, dissertations and specialist books.

Visit us on the internet:

http://www.grin.com/

http://www.facebook.com/grincom

http://www.twitter.com/grin_com

IMPLEMENTATION OF THE WARD BASED OUTREACH TEAMS PROGRAMME IN THE RURAL AREA OF KGETLENG SUB-DISTRICT, NORTH WEST PROVINCE.

By

MR. RODNEY AZWINNDINI MULELU

Ellisras Hospital
Department of Health
Limpopo Province
Lephalale

Theme: 'Interdisciplinary Approaches to sustainability Accounting and Management'
(The role of Sustainability accounting on the new UN Sustainable Development Goals [SDGS]).

ABSTRACT

This paper investigates the implementation of ward Based Outreach Teams programme in the rural areas of the Kgetleng sub district, in the North West Province of South Africa. The Department of Health has set a long-term goal of establishing National Health Insurance in the country. This would provide equitable and universal coverage for a defined package of healthcare. One of the key pillars of National Health Insurance is the re-engineering of Primary Health Care, which has at its heart in the development of Ward-Based Outreach Teams who will take the responsibility for specific groups of households.

In this regard, the South African Department of Health has considered re-engineering of the Primary Health Care model in the country in making sure health resources; technology and quality services are available, accessible and affordable to all communities. The North West province Department of Health is currently piloting the Primary Health Care re-engineering programme, which include the Ward Based Outreach Teams programme in all four Districts. Bojanala, Ngaka Modiri Molema, Dr. Kenneth Kaunda and Dr Ruth Segomotsi Mompati. In Bojanala District, the pilot site is in ward five in Kgetleng sub district.

In this paper, the quantitative research design was used where self – administered questionnaires were provided to the Community Health Workers (CHW) and the Outreach team leaders (OTL) for data collection. The findings of the paper indicated that Ward Based Outreach Teams contribute towards a better understanding of local health care needs, inform service priorities, refer patients to different stakeholders, and build stronger relationships between service providers and users in the communities. The key elements to practice this service are person-centred comprehensive care, collaboration between people, practitioners, and continuity of health care in the community.

Key words: Ward Based Outreach Teams (WBOT), Primary Health Care (PHC), Community Health Workers (CHW), Outreach Team Leaders (OTL), District Management Team (DMT) and PHC re-engineering

TABLE OF CONTENTS

1. INTRODUCTION 3
2. BACKGROUND TO THE PAPER 3
3. STATEMENT OF THE RESEARCH PROBLEM 4
4. RESEARCH METHODOLOGY 4
5. LITERATURE REVIEW 5
   5.1. WARD BASED OUTREACH TEAMS (WBOT) PROGRAMME IN SOUTH AFRICA 5
   5.2. KEY ASPECTS OF COMPREHENSIVE PHC IMPLEMENTATION 6
   5.3. FACTORS THAT FACILITATE SUCCESS OF WBOT IMPLEMENTATION 7
6. LESSONS LEARNED FROM INTERNATIONAL EXPERIENCES 7
   6.1. LESSONS LEARNED FROM CUBA 7
   6.2. LESSONS LEARNED FROM BRAZIL 7
   6.3. LESSON LEARNED FROM ZAMBIA 8
7. DISCUSSION OF THE FINDINGS 9
8. CONCLUSIONS FROM THE FINDINGS 10
9. RECOMMENDATIONS 12
10. CONCLUSION 12
REFERENCES 13

1. INTRODUCTION

According to Bam, Marcus and Hugo[1] South Africa has established ward-based Community Health Workers (CHW) outreach teams, as part of a series of strategies to strengthen primary health care. The key elements to practice this service are person-centered comprehensive care, collaboration between people, practitioners, and continuity of health care. This will be community-orientated primary healthcare (COPC) on a massive scale, and it is estimated that 7 000 such teams all over the country (Community Health Workers and a nurse, supported by a doctor) need to be established. They would provide basic preventive care and health promotion, identify people at risk, support adherence in chronic care, offer home-based care and help integrate care at the community level (Mash and Blitz, [2].

WBOTs in the local areas are supported by a PHC clinic that is largely nurse-driven, with part-time support from a doctor. In overall support of these WBOTs and clinics, a family physician is required to ensure evidence-based best practice, integrate care, help evaluate and reflect on what is happening, as well as mentor and capacitate team members. This research will be an important contributor to achieving these goals (Beasley, Starfield, van Weel, Rosser and Haq [3]. The delivery of the health system in South Africa and other developing countries is an important measure that affects a country's health status (Marmot, Ryff, Bumpass, Shipley and Marks, [4]. The healthcare service delivery system is the mode to combine inputs and to allow the delivery of a series of interventions or serviced actions in order to improve the health condition of people (Bhattacharyya, McGahan, Dunne, Singer and Daar [5]. This study investigated the implementation of the Ward Based Outreach Teams (WBOT) in a rural area in the Kgetleng Sub-district, North West Province.

2. BACKGROUND TO THE PAPER

According to Motsieng [6], the MEC for the Department of Health in the North West Province has indicated that in the 2012/2013 financial year, the WBOT programme will make the financial year a defining moment in the history of the health service delivery in the North West Province. In addition, Outreach Teams (WBOT) will soon be on the ground visiting patients in their homes and providing the much needed health care services. "The WBOT approach will require all of us as health professionals, tribal authorities, the community, various families and patients themselves to work together to fight diseases from inside of our homes and out in broader communities", said Dr. Masike(Motsieng,[6].

However, in light of all discussed above, the health sector in the province, in South Africa and in developing countries are still faced with so many challenges. These challenges are the huge health status gap between urban and rural areas, low level of health awareness, cost of healthcare, scarcity of specialty care and under-resourced infrastructure (Schneider & Barron, [7]. In recent years, these health sector problems have become more serious and higher priority has been given to delivering health service and meeting the needs of the poor in rural areas in many countries (Reddy, Patel and Jha, [8].

It is recognized and indicated that strengthening health delivery system as a priority for countries and governments to be able to meet the basic health needs of their people, especially for poor and vulnerable populations (Marmot, Allen and Bell, [9]). Challenges in the province and developing countries, including South Africa, are to find ways which will enable to address this basic health needs more effectively (David, Sameh, Banafsheh, Katja and Marko, [10].

3. STATEMENT OF THE RESEARCH PROBLEM

The Kgetleng Sub-district is one of the pilot projects since the Ward Based Outreach Teams (WBOTs) programme was first established in the Bojanala District in North West Province in 2011. This is one of the three areas of the PHC re-engineering strategy being implemented in the Province of the North-West and the rest of the country.

Department of Health, [11] indicates that there are high rates of maternal death, defaulters and lost to follow-up of patients on HIV and TB medication. These are the challenges that face the Kgetleng sub-district in the optimal implementation of the WBOT programme in the district.

The problem the paper is focused on, therefore, was to gain insight into the understanding of the implementation of the Ward Based Outreach Teams (WBOT) programme in the rural areas of Kgetleng Sub-district, in the North-West Province.

4. RESEARCH METHODOLOGY

The research design that is applied in this paper is descriptive. A quantitative research method was used. Quantitative methodology is associated with analytical research and its purpose is to arrive at a universal statement. Leedy & Ormrod, [12] point out that a quantitative method begins with a series of predetermined categories, usually embodied in standardised measures and uses these data to make broad and general comparisons. The quantitative method was based primarily on confidentially structured questionnaires provided to 27 Community Health Workers.

The Kgetleng Sub-district has 41 CHWs (Department of Health, [11]). The target population for this paper was CHWs working at the WBOT in the rural area of the Kgetleng Sub-district. In this paper, the population consisted of Kgetleng Community Health Workers (24), Outreach Team Leaders (2), and Professional nurse (1) of the feeder clinic. Twenty seven (27) respondents make up the paper population. These respondents resided within the catchment area of the Kgetleng Sub-district.

Self-administered questionnaires have been used for the purpose of this paper. The development of a questionnaire was informed by reading and reviewing of the literature during proposal writing. A total number of twenty seven (27) questionnaires were distributed to the targeted respondents. The use of self-administered questionnaires in the data collection process is critical, since it makes large samples feasible and has an important strength with regard to measurement generally (Leedy and Ormrod,[13].

Leedy and Ormrod, [14] state that data analysis in a case paper involves the steps listed below:

- Organisation of detail about the case – the specific facts about the case is arranged in a logical order.
- Categorisations of data – categories are identified to help cluster the data into meaningful groups.
- Interpretation of patterns – specific documents, occurrences, and other bits of data are examined for the specific meaning that they might have in relation to the case.
- Identification of patterns – the data and their interpretations are scrutinized for underlying themes and other patterns that characterize the case more broadly than a single piece of information can reveal.
- Synthesis and generalization – conclusions are drawn that may have implication beyond the specific case that has been studied.

In this particular paper, data analysis followed a quantitative research analysis approach and steps mentioned above for data obtained through the questionnaires.

5. LITERATURE REVIEW

The Department of Health has embarked on a strategy for re-modelling the implementation of the primary health care system using community and clinical health care worker teams to improve support and to strengthen the districts health services. Primary Health Care re-engineering has three streams: Ward Based Outreach Teams (WBOT), District Clinical Specialist Teams (DCST) and the School Health Programme. The integration and collaboration across all three streams is important to ensure the improvement and success of the primary health care across the district and the Province of the North West and to improve maternal and child health outcomes (NDOH, [15].

5.1. WARD BASED OUTREACH TEAMS (WBOT) PROGRAMME IN SOUTH AFRICA

According to Sepulveda [16], observations from many developing countries suggest that provision of home and community based health services and their links with the fixed PHC facilities in particular are critical to good health outcomes, especially child health outcomes. The role of community health workers in many countries has contributed to better health outcomes (WHO, [17].

The South African Department of Health has suggested that this is the result of a multiplicity of factors related to community based health workers. The adverse factors include inadequate training, inadequate support and supervision, random distribution with poor coverage, no link between the communities based services and services offered by fixed health facilities, funding through NGOs with inadequate accountability, limited or no targets for either coverage or quality to be reached (NDOH, [18]. According to Friis-Hannsen and Cold-Ravnkilde, [19] the impact of HIV on key impact indicators has also contributed considerably to the relatively poor health indicators and is independent of interventions made by CHWs or other health workers and interventions.

Many of these factors could be corrected if CHWs were part of a team, were well trained, supported and supervised with a clear mandate both in terms of what they are expected to do and of the catchment population that they are responsible for. The ward based PHC outreach team is designed to correct these limitations in the way community based health services are currently provided in the country (Gemma, [20]).

Given the key role that CHWs will play, they should, over time, be directly managed by the Department of Health (as opposed to NGOs). This move has already happened in all the provinces in the country. The strategies for direct management by the Department have already happened and all the districts in the country have done an audit on the number of CHWs, to be trained and employed by the Department of Health as CHWs. The PHC reengineering toolkit for implementation of the WBOT in provinces indicates that each team is linked to a PHC facility with a nurse in each facility, who is the team leader.

The team leader is responsible for ensuring that their work is targeted and linked to service delivery targets and that they are adequately supported and supervised – this approach has been adopted and provinces have been implementing this strategy as from 2011 (NDOH, 2011, Matsoso and Fryatt, [18]-[21]. The WBOT implementation tool kit also indicates that the re-engineered approach to providing PHC services proposes a population based approach for the delivery of services. In addition, the PHC outreach is a service to the uninsured population of South Africa.

It further indicates that the Department of Health in a sub-district or on local levels will deploy PHC outreach teams in rural areas, in informal urban settlements as well as townships. According to Matsoso and Fryatt, [21], the Ward Based PHC Outreach Teams (WBOT) which are one of the one streams of the re-engineered PHC model are the level of health service which provides services to communities, families and individuals at community – based institutions and at a household level in a ward.

Furthermore, the ward based PHC outreach team is the cornerstone of community based PHC services, which encompass activities in communities, households and educational institutions, and referral networks with community based providers. The researcher, however, will only concentrate on and conducts this research on the Ward Based Outreach Teams (WBOT) area of PHC reengineering.

The diagrammatic PHC Outreach Teams (WBOT) model is presented in figure 2.1 below.

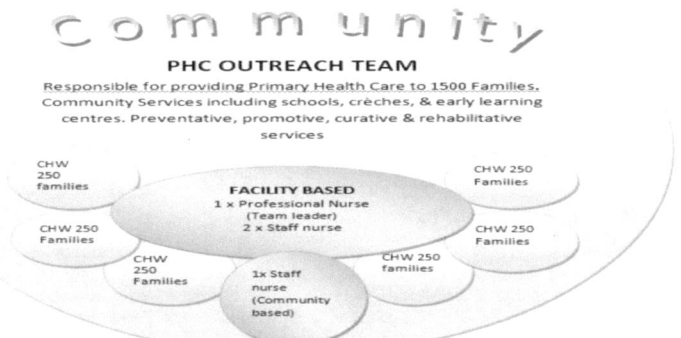

FIGURE 2.1: THE WARD BASED PRIMARY HEALTH CARE OUTREACH TEAM (WBOT) ADAPTED FROM NDOH (2011)

5.2. KEY ASPECTS OF COMPREHENSIVE PHC IMPLEMENTATION

The WHO, [22] indicates eight elements that form the basis of comprehensive PHC programme interventions in order to achieve the goal of health improvement. These elements include the following: "education on prevailing health problems and methods of preventing and controlling them; promotion of food supply and proper nutrition; an adequate supply of safe water and basic sanitation; maternal and child health care including family planning, immunization against major infectious diseases; appropriate treatment of common diseases and injuries; and the provision of essential drugs." (Lehmann and Sanders, [23].

Denhill, King and Swanepoel, [24] indicate that, overall, in any health care programme or strategy, the successful implementation of PHC must be guided by the following principles:

- Political will: The presence of progressive political will is central to the success of a health system.
- Integration of promotive, curative, preventive and rehabilitative health care services.
- Equity: Communities must have equal access to basic health care and social services without segregation of sub-groups and provision of care.
- Accessibility: Health services must reach all people in the country in terms of geographical, financial and functional accessibility.
- Affordability: The level of health care services must be in line with what the community and country can afford. Not being able to afford should not be a limiting factor to receiving health care.
- Availability: An adequate and appropriate health services to meet particular health needs of each community.
- Effectiveness: Health services provided must meet the objectives for which they were intended and should be justifiable in terms of funding.
- Efficiency: Objectives and goals accomplished should be balanced to resources used.

These principles mentioned above determine the success or failure of any WBOT and PHC programme worldwide.

5.3. FACTORS THAT FACILITATE SUCCESS OF WBOT IMPLEMENTATION

Most comprehensive PHC programmes that are successful come as a result of good government policies and legislature for equitable implementation of efficient and furthermore, cost-effective health care interventions emphasize the need for community and individual participation according to Lewin and Lehmann, [25].

- Government commitment and will
- Community participation by stakeholders
- Cost-effectiveness, efficiencies and equity

6. LESSONS LEARNED FROM INTERNATIONAL EXPERIENCES

6.1. LESSONS LEARNED FROM CUBA

According to Gorry and Keck, [26], Cuba is an example of the successful implementation of community participation. It involved the integration of the mass democratic movement into formal governance structures, including health. Institutional structures were developed to allow for the participation of communities in decision making and policy processes. Furthermore, public officials were elected to People Power Assemblies at the provincial and national level to represent community interests. In addition, all authority comes from the people and all accountability comes from the state to the people according to Birkland [27].

Oviedo, [28] state that, In Cuba, Each People Power Assembly at each level of government appoints the personnel of the administrative agencies assigned to it. Each health facility had an advisory committee consisting of representatives; management consults with the advisory committee on issues that affect or require participation from the community. Though rarely done, the community has the power to request the removal of health workers. In addition, Cuba developed a unique Family Doctor Programme that attaches a family doctor and a nurse to every 120-140 families. These health workers are responsible for all the health needs of that community (including health education, promotion and curative services). Furthermore, this has strengthened communities' understanding of health matters, and promoted the collective discussion and solution of health problems, thereby improving the families and communities' participatory skills. However, a criticism of this approach is that it fostered dependence on medical interventions of the communities.

6.2. LESSONS LEARNED FROM BRAZIL

According to Spink, [29], the example of the Unified Health System in Brazil has been the guiding vision behind the South African Re-engineering Policy. Furthermore, social participation in health is mandated by the constitution to be included in all levels of government (Health councils – 1 national, 27 state and 5500 municipal).

According to Crisp, [30] the health councils are permanent bodies in charge of formulating health strategies, controlling implementation of policies, and analysing health plans and management reports submitted by their respective level of government. Furthermore, strong interactions exist between councils, managers, and policy makers, forming a complex and innovative decision-making process. All councils are made up of health care users (50% of members), health workers (25%), and health managers and service providers (25%).

In addition, health conferences are held every four years at the three levels. The mandate of these conferences is to assess the health situation and propose directives for health policies, thus contributing to inclusion of themes in the public agenda. Among other democratic mechanisms, the participatory budget adopted by several states and municipalities is also innovative. A proportion of the health budget for a city (municipality) or state is defined on the basis of popular vote; the population of a given city can vote, for example, on whether a new intensive-care unit or more health posts should be built according to Crisp, [29].

6.3. LESSON LEARNED FROM ZAMBIA

According to Resnick, [30], declining Gross Domestic Product (GDP) and decreasing health budgets have impacted negatively on many countries in Africa. In Zambia, for instance, PHC implementation began in August 1981, with steady progress and interventions that included the training of community health workers, construction and upgrading of rural health centers, improved distribution of medicine, a strengthened transport system, as well as improved health planning and management.

Furthermore, these interventions were largely driven by the economic boost that Zambia experienced due to the increase in the global demand for copper - Zambia's main export product and the country's major source of income at the time according to Resnick, [31]. Furthermore, the current public health system is two-tiered as well as inequitable and unsustainable in terms of poor financial resources allocation, inadequate human resource, staff turnover and unequal access to health care services.

The two-tiered system is characterized by poor management, supervision and poor quality of health care services and deteriorating infrastructure in the public sector, whilst the private sector is characterized by over-pricing of services (Kautzky et al, [32]. The next section will discuss the findings of the study from the data collected.

7. DISCUSSION OF THE FINDINGS

Question: 1. what are the challenges and successes that you experienced with examples and give your views of the WBOT programme?

All 100% respondents indicated challenges and successes encountered with WBOT programme. The respondents indicated that they worked hard in spite of the challenges to achieve the WBOT goals and objectives. However, there are also successes with this programme such as many patients are able to adhere to treatment and live their healthy lives. The responses also indicated that there are challenges and successes in the WBOT programme.

The challenges are such as patients not wanting the CHWs to know their status, early booking of anti-natal clinic, adherence to antiretroviral (ARV) regime, shortage of vitamin A or patients giving wrong addresses. However, there are successes in the programme such as patients being able to be referred to the clinic for treatment early or the community being able to get knowledge on different diseases in a form of one on one and campaigns. Nxumalo and Choonara, [33] state the importance of mobilizing, communicating with and involving local stakeholders including Department of Health to generate support and develop networks that can continue to support WBOT to address the challenges highlighted above.

Question 2: Respondents knowledge of factors that make the implementation of the WBOT programme a success/failure.

In this section, the researcher discusses the factors mentioned by respondents that make the implementation of the WBOT programme a success or failure. All 100% respondents' indicated that they have difficulties when referring patients to the clinics. One respondent indicated that "some nurses are rude to the patients when they refer patients to nurses." This results in patients refusing to go to the clinic when referred. They indicated that they are unable to provide patients in the community optimal support due to poor participation of so community structures.

Negative attitude towards the respondents by the community and the nurses in the clinics were also indicated in this study as a factor in the success of WBOT programme.
Furthermore, respondents indicated that community structures are not involved and recommended that they need to be encouraged, allow them to be fully involved and participate in health issues. From the responses, it is found that community participation and negative attitudes in health issues of some structures and nurses are some of the factors that contribute to the WBOT programme success or failure.

Question 3: What are the difficulties of working with nurses in the health facilities?

All 100% respondents had different forms of difficulties working with nurses in the facilities. Difficulties such as bad attitude, not taking us (CHWs) seriously, not completing the referral forms, not wanting to touch the patients because of bad smell were major difficulties indicated by respondents in working with nurses in the facilities.
It is clear that there are difficulties in working with nurses in the health facilities. Respondents indicated that some nurses are being rude to the patients when they referred to the facility, this results in patients refusing to go to the clinic when referred. Nxumalo and Choonara, [33] highlight the importance of working with all stakeholders including nurses for optimal implementation of the WBOT programme.

Question 4: What are the benefits of working with nurses and patients in the health facilities?

All 100% respondents indicated the benefits of working with nurses and patients in the health facilities. The respondents indicated that some nurses do co-operate and help us by talking to patients in a correct manner. They make things easy for us and the patients. Regarding the patients, they indicated that they become impossible, refusing to take treatment, and even to go to the clinic for admissions.

It came out that despite the difficulties working with nurses; there are benefits of working with the nurses in the facilities. According to Nxumalo et al, [33], it is indicated that working hand in hand with the government, the community structures, nurses and patients is critical in the success of WBOT programme. It has been shown in these responses that working together with nurses will improve the programme.

Question 5: What strategies are there to improve community participation?

All 100% respondents indicated that there are challenges that are facing community structures with WBOT and also highlighted the strategies that can improve community participation in the WBOT programme. They indicated that it is important for all relevant structures and stakeholders to meet and plan together; otherwise the community would not be able to attend these meetings. They also indicated that the community is tired by meetings and campaigns that are coordinated separately without its involvement. It is noted in the survey that community mobilization and involving local stakeholders to generate support is critical.

According to Dennill et al, [24], community participation is a critical support activity for PHC system to achieve the goal of health for all. The responses in the table 5 above indicate that respondents are in agreement that there are challenges that the community structures are facing to encourage and support WBOT. Some of those challenges are: the Department of Health does not listen to the community needs, the feedback is not taken seriously, and there is a great need for educating the community and their leaders in terms of WBOT. It came out clearly in these responses, that stakeholder involvement and participation is a key in the success of the WBOT programme.

8. CONCLUSIONS FROM THE FINDINGS

The results from the respondents have shown that there are successes, challenges and lesson learned from this paper. The results of the paper indicate that the programme is being implemented well even though it is in its pilot phase in the sub-district. It has shown that more and more people are being helped by CHWs in their own homes. The long queues in the clinics have been reduced, because many patients are treated at home by the CHWs. The programme has managed to improve and it saves many lives in the communities of the Kgetleng Sub-district.

In addition, the findings of the paper also indicated challenges such as bad attitude of some nurses in the facilities, nurses not able to complete the referral forms, wrong addresses by patients and refusal of some patients to allow the CHWs to visit and enter their homes. Furthermore, the findings of this survey highlighted the importance of mobilizing and involving local stakeholders to generate support. They also can develop networks that can continue to support WBOT implementation.

Objective 1: To evaluate the experiences of CHWs in the implementation of the WBOT programme.

The findings showed that respondents regarded WBOT as a good programme and as one that is doing well. Experiences by CHWs such as unwillingness of the patients to disclose their status, giving wrong addresses, patients swearing at the CHWs, lack of knowledge of the community regarding WBOT, and finally, a lack of community participation were found to hamper the successes of the programme. However, willingness and commitment to help the community from the CHWs enhanced the WBOT programme implementation. Despite challenges that the CHWs experienced in their duties, they continued working and helping the community to be a better and healthier one.

According to the WHO, [22], community participation is a critical support activity for the PHC system to achieve the goal of health for all. In addition, participation should be active, communities have the right and responsibility to exercise power over the decisions that affect their lives and there must be mechanisms to allow for the implementation of the decisions by the community (Dennil et al, [24].

The findings for the paper indicated that there are still challenges regarding optimal community participation in the health issues in the community. One respondent indicated that "when they organize campaigns, some people don't attend, so the information is not spreading as it should'. Furthermore, the findings indicated in this paper that the referral system is a big challenge for the respondents when conducting their work. According to WHO, [17], a referral system plays one of the key roles and gives input to the approach for the optimal implementation of the WBOT programme.
In addition, the CHWs role in the household is to assess and identify health problems in the community, and if needs be, refer to the nearest facility. According to the NDOH, [18], referral forms should be completed by the Outreach Team Leader (OTL) to the clinic and the clinic to the Outreach Team. However, this is not the case

according to the respondents. They encounter problems of nurses not completing the back referral form and they indicate that this causes the patients to default.

The findings from this objective is a clear indication that CHWs, community structures, all stakeholders should be supported, planning together with government entities and ward counselors in the community would achieve the desired goals that will help the community to get more involved in the WBOT programme.

Objective 2: To identify and evaluate factors that facilitates the implementation of the WBOT programme

The section on factors facilitating the implementation of the WBOT programme have shown that working hand in hand with the community structures, ward counsellors and the nurses in the clinics is critical to the success of the WBOT programme. Of the 12 respondents, eleven (92%) share their views of what they encounter from the community regarding the WBOT programme. However, one (8%) of the respondents felt that as CHWs, they are not being taken seriously.

Nxumalo and Choonara, [33], in their rapid assessment of the WBOT programme findings, highlight the importance of mobilizing and involving local stakeholders to generate support and also develop networks that can continue to support the WBOT programme implementation. The findings of this paper further indicated all twelve (100%) respondents encounter some form of difficulties with nurses when working in the health facilities.

The difficulties mentioned by the respondents are (but not limited to): bad attitude, being rude to patients, failure to record after issuing medication, not being taken seriously, nurses not completing the back referral form, not wanting to touch the patients because of a bad smell. These were major difficulties that the respondents encountered when working with the nurses and they indicated that they sometimes compel the patients in the household not interested to go to the health facility (clinic) when referred.

However, there are also benefits of working with nurses in the health facilities. The respondent number one (1) indicated that "*some nurses are cooperative and help us by talking to the patients in a correct manner and they even fill out the back referral forms*". Respondent number three (3) indicated that nurses are knowledgeable in the field of health and are able to give advice; and where they are not competent, they refer to the medical officer.

Objective 3: To make recommendations to the District Management Team with regards to the findings of the paper to be implemented.

The respondents suggested various strategies and recommendations to improve the WBOT programme implementation. All 100% respondents suggested that they needed support beyond the normal duties that they conduct in the communities, such as taken seriously and be appointed permanently as government workers. Suggestions for improvements included:

- Local stakeholders in the community to meet, plan and coordinate together
- Improve mobilization and involving local stakeholders
- Training and education of the community about WBOT
- Strengthen communication amongst the community structures and
- Conducting community campaigns and dialogues so that the community can understand WBOT and get involved.

9. RECOMMENDATIONS

The next section will outline the recommendations of the paper for various stakeholders in WBOT programme.

It is recommended that:

- The North West Department of Health should recruit more male CHWs for gender representations in the community structure making males to see the contribution they can make in the WBOT programme. There is a need to formulate a gender mainstreaming policy on hiring of CHWs in this programme. Information on all aspects of CHWs appointment criteria should be known to all members of community.
- Department of Health in the North West should recruit more CHWs under the age of 40 years because they are still young and able to cover the long distance walking.
- The respondents ought to be trained and to be provided with career pathing. The CHWs have been provided with Phase 1 training and are still to continue to Phase 2 training and Phase 3 NQF qualifications, which is a one year occupational training accredited by QCTO; finishing this they would be able to enter into health promotion field. The Department of Health in the North West should continue to recruit more OTL and CHWs to cover all the wards needed for optimal implementation of the WBOT programme.
- Professional development and mentoring opportunities for CHWs and the OTLs should be provided, as many of them have a working service of between 1- 3 years.
- A conducive working environment should be created by providing good working relationships with providers of service such nurses, social workers, health promotion and environmental health practitioners to respond to needs of the communities.
- Policy changes need to be communicated efficiently, both to health professionals and the community to avoid resistance and confusion.

10. CONCLUSION

This paper indicates that the successful WBOT programme provides a more holistic approach to addressing the health needs of all individuals and promotes the development of community participation, provision of staff in clinics that have positive attitudes and willing to help the community. In addition, this paper shows that proper referral system, working together with stakeholders is important for smooth running of the WBOT programme in the community. In addition, resources are needed to support CHWs; these are cadres that help people who are sick in the community. Furthermore, this paper shows that CHWs can make a valuable contribution to community health development and more specifically, they can improve access to and coverage of communities with basic health services.

REFERENCES

1. Bam, N. (2013). Conceptualizing community oriented primary care (COPC)--the Tshwane, South Africa, health post model. *African Journal of Primary Health Care & Family Medicine*, 3-7.
2. Mash, R. (2015). Overcoming challenges in primary care education in South Africa. Education for Primary Care, 274-278.
3. Beasley, JW, Starfield B, van Weel C, Rosser WW & Haq CL. (2007). Global health and primary care research. J Am Board Fam Med 20(6):518-526. Available at: http://dx.doi.org/10.3122/jabfm.2007.06.070172. Accessed 10 June 2015
4. Marmot M, Ryff CD, Bumpass LL, Shipley M & Marks NF. (1997). Social inequalities in health: next questions and converging evidence, Soc Sci Med, 44, 901-10
5. Bhattacharyya, O, McGahan A, Dunne D, Singer PA & Daar A. (2008). Innovative Health Service Delivery Models for Low and Middle Income Countries, the Rockefeller Foundation, Washington.
6. Motsieng, N (2012). Primary Health care Revamp. Piloting of NHI. Boitekanelo, April – June, P6-8.
7. Schneider H & Barron P. (2008). Achieving the Millennium Development Goals in South Africa through the revitalization of primary health care and a strengthened District health system, Position paper, University of Cape Town.
8. Reddy, KS. (2011). Towards achievement of universal health care in India by 2020: a call to action. The Lancet , 760-768.
9. Marmot, M. (2012). WHO European review of social determinants of health and the health divide. The Lancet , 1011-1029.
10. David, HP, Sameh E, Banafsheh S, Katja J & Marko V. (2009). Improving Health Service Delivery in Developing Countries, the World Bank, Washington, DC, 978-08213-7888-5.
11. Department of Health (2015). Bojanala District services. North West Province. District Annual Performance Reports, 2014/15 .
12. Leedy, PD & Ormrod, JE. (2012). Practical Research Planning and Design. Ninth Edition. Always learning. Pearson Publishers
13. Leedy, PD & Ormrod, JE. (2013). Practical Research Planning and Design. Tenth Edition. Always learning. Pearson Publishers
14. Leedy, PD & Ormrod, JE. (2014). Practical Research Planning and Design. Eleventh Edition. Always learning. Pearson Publishers
15. NDOH, (2012). South Africa. Case paper: Integrating the three streams of PHC Re-engineering: Establishing the link between the school health barriers, teams and DCST in Lejweleputswa District, Free State.
16. Sepulveda J, Bustreo F &Tapia R. (2006). Improvement of child survival in Mexico: the diagonal approach. The Lancet, 368, pp 2017-2027.
17. WHO, (2007). Community health workers: What do we know about them? The state of the evidence on programmes, activities, costs and impact on health outcomes of using community health workers. WHO Evidence and Information for Policy, Department of Human Resources for Health, Geneva. January 2007.
18. NDOH, (2011). South Africa. Provincial Guidelines for the Implementation of the Three Streams of PHC Re-engineering. Republic of South Africa: Department of Health. 4 September 2011.
19. Friis-Hansen, E. (2013). Social accountability mechanisms and access to public service delivery in rural Africa. DIIS Reports, Danish Institute for International Studies.
20. Gemma, R. (2015). Review of the evidence for adolescent and young person specific, community-based health services for NHS managers. Journal of Children's Services, 57-75.
21. Matsoso, MP. (2012). National Health Insurance: the first 18 months: legislation and financing. South African Health Review , 21-33.
22. WHO, (2014). The World Health Report 2014: Primary health care (now more than ever).
23. Lehmann U & Sanders D. (2007). Community Health Workers: what do we know about them? http://www.who.int/hrh/documents/community_health_workers.pdf Accessed 8 June 2015.
24. Dennill, K, King, L & Swanepol, T. (1998). Aspects of primary health care; community health care in Southern Africa. Oxford University Press, Southern Africa: Cape Town.
25. Lewin, S. (2013). Governing Large-Scale Community Health Worker Programs. 3-4.
26. Gorry, C. (2014). The Cuban Health System. A Contemporary Cuba Reader: The Revolution under Raul Castro , 407.
27. Birkland, TA. (2014). An introduction to the policy process: Theories, concepts and models of public policy making. New york. Routledge.
28. Oviedo, E. (2011). e-Health in Latin America and the Caribbean: progress and challenges. ECLAC. Available at http//www.repositorio.cepal.org. Accessed 25 November 2015.
29. Spink, P. (2011). Innovations in Government from around the World: the most recent awards winners from the Ford Foundation sponsored Innovations Programs in Brazil, Chile, China, and East.
30. Crisp, N. (2014). HIV/AIDS and National Health Insurance in South Africa. African Health Leaders: Making Change and Claiming the Future , 249.
31. Resnick, D. (2014). The Political Economy of Zambia's Recovery: Structural Change without Transformation. IFPRI Discussion Paper 01320.
32. Kautzky, K & Tollman, SM. (2009). A perspective on primary health care in South Africa. Health Systems Trust: South Africa.
33. Nxumalo, N & Choonara, S. (2014). Ward – Based Community Health Worker Outreach Teams: The success of Sedibeng Health Posts. The Centre for Health Policy (CHP), Health policy and system Research. Policy brief. Wits University.

YOUR KNOWLEDGE HAS VALUE

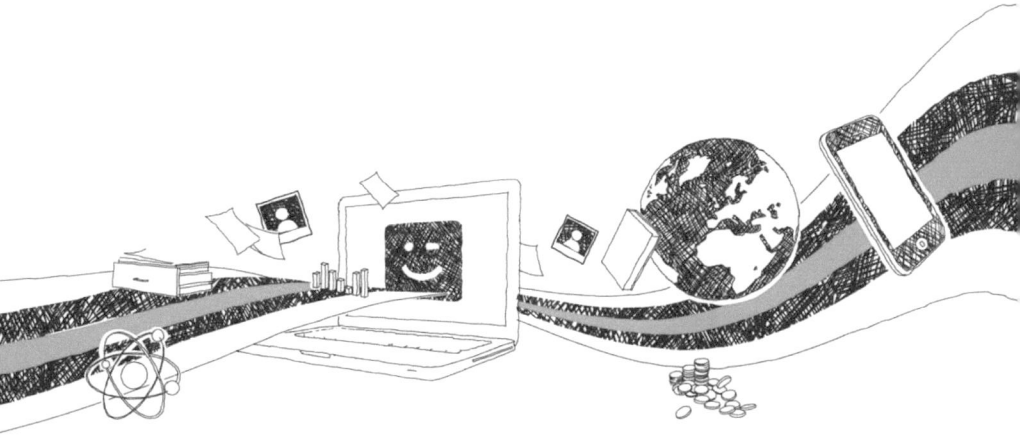

- We will publish your bachelor's and master's thesis, essays and papers

- Your own eBook and book - sold worldwide in all relevant shops

- Earn money with each sale

Upload your text at www.GRIN.com
and publish for free

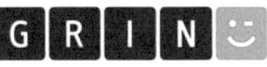